Fat Girl Pick Your Head Up

AHLUMBA HARRIS

To order additional copies of this book, contact:

Inspired2Prosper International LLC
contactus@inspired2prosper.com
www.inspired2prosper.com
www.ahlumba.com

DEDICATION

To all those who dreamed a dream that seemed impossible I implore you to keep going. Your gift was given to you for a reason, so don't allow it to remain dormant due to fear, lack or uncertainty.

CONTENTS

ACKNOWLEDGMENTS

To someone very special; I thank you for loving all the versions of me: the fat girl, the skinny girl, the ugly girl, the pretty girl, the insecure girl, the mean girl, and most of all the emotional girl. Aniyla; you are an extension of me and I will always and forever love you! To my family you all rock (some more than others) one hundred times over you all inspire me.

A special thank you to the men and woman who believed enough in my gift to step out on faith by planting a financial seed into my gift and ultimately helped to make it possible for me to continue making my dream a reality: *Kimberly Hill, Gerald Middlebrooks, Wesley Bradley, Tionna Davis, Gibran and Christie Harris.*

Can't Stop Seeking It's Approval

My scale hates me
Yet I can't seem to let it go
Constantly It shows me numbers
That I don't want to know
Daily I say
One day I will let it go
But it calls back to me
By way of my tight fitting clothes
My scale hates me
Yet I refuse to let it go
Cause I know that one day
It will tell me what I want to know
~Ahlumba

Chapter
1

FORCED TO LOOK IN THE MIRROR

My Story/What Started It All

Shame, insecurity, loneliness, sadness, isolation, unpretty, and fat were some of the words that most accurately described the emotions I felt towards myself on a daily basis. I was 5'2, weighed a whopping 195, pounds and all I could wonder was, "How did this happen? How did I become what I always said I would never be?"

As a child and leading up to my teens, weight was never an issue. It was not until I left home, had the freedom of my own money, and the ability to use it as I chose that I slowly began to gain weight. The lack of restriction that came with being on my own was wonderful. I was grown, no longer had my parents ruling over me, and could eat whatever I wanted. So, I became a takeout junkie. I ate in excess all of the things that were to long denied me as a child. Slowly, the buildup of my unhealthy bad eating began to have and show its negative effects on my body.

Within six months I went from weighing 125 pounds to weighing 150 pounds. Though I noticed the outward change showed to me by the scale I still did not rein in my eating. Until eventually I began to hear comments such as, *"Are you gaining weight?"* Yes, I was gaining weight, but I still looked good and had a flat stomach so I kept it moving, ignored their comments, and continued eating the same way.

Then it happened, about five months before I was to turn twenty, something life changing occurred...I found out that I was pregnant. During that pregnancy I gained an additional thirty pounds, which when added to the twenty-five that I had already gained previously was quite a considerable amount. Young and full of myself - I was somewhat unmoved by the additional pounds for I arrogantly thought the weight would come off quick and easy, apparently so easy without even the need of any exercise.

After giving birth to my daughter I weighed about 180 pounds, which included what I like to call "my freshman twenty five" that I gained from being on my own, and then the added thirty pounds from the pregnancy. To my delight, I was able to lose some of the baby weight, which enabled me to stuff myself back into at least one pair of my pre-maternity jeans. However after dropping those initial ten pounds I gained it back plus more. Leaving me at a consistent weight of 195 pounds - the biggest I had ever been in my life.

Unsure and unhappy with myself, I turned into the mean fat girl that no one liked, until the day came that I was finally forced to look at the person I had become. What I saw I did not recognize nor did I like.

SO IT BEGINS

Being overweight is no fairytale; I cannot truthfully say that it was a struggle, for I was too lazy to put forth the effort to do the necessary work needed to get the weight off. On most occasions I spent my time trying to find fast and easy ways to lose the extra weight I had gained.

Out of desperation and laziness I tried several products and fad diets that I thought would help me to lose the excessive weight quickly. For example: pills, not eating, grapefruit juice, ect… To help you to better understand the true extent of my laziness I will break it down for you one-by-one:

1. **Pills:** One day, I decided to visit a vitamin store to inquire about some weight loss pills, and Hydroxycut was recommended (back in early 2000 Hydroxycut was a very popular weight loss supplement). Needless to say I purchased them. However after two or three days of using the pills I stopped. I had begun to notice my heart beating in a very irregular way and decided that I was not trying to get sick - just to lose weight. I never

touched pills again.

2. **Not Eating:** Obviously something I was putting in my mouth was causing all this weight gain. Though I was partially correct I chose to go about correcting it in a totally incorrect manner. I thought starvation was the key. But, of course, my resolve to starve never lasted long. As soon as the hunger pains racked my body I would always eat in the end.

3. **Salad:** I have always enjoyed salads so when I tried to make the choice to eat nothing but salad everyday (what a joke that was) not only did I not have the budget, I also lacked the determination, and of course it turned out not to be a healthy diet nor a proper way to lose weight.

4. **Grapefruit Juice:** I cannot believe that I thought I could lose over fifty pounds by just drinking grapefruit juice...Enough said.

5. **Vinegar:** I was told that apple cider vinegar burned fat and that if I took a tablespoon of apple cider vinegar before every meal it would help me lose my weight. Now maybe that does work when one is eating in a proper manner, however, I was not. I laugh now when I think of it, because for me to think that I would lose weight just from drinking vinegar was equivalent to me thinking that I could supersize a meal and balance it out by ordering a diet coke.

6. **Enlisting in the Army:** At my absolute lowest I considered joining the Army. One day while looking at the television a commercial came on about Army boot-camp and I thought *maybe they can get me into shape* but thankfully I got a hold of my senses for at least a brief moment to realize that this was a ridiculous idea.

There I was, expending all this energy on easy ways to lose weight; yet the one necessary obvious constant I continued to deliberately allow myself to exclude and elude was exercise. After about five years of complaining about my weight, wishing I would lose it, and avoiding mirrors so that I did not have to see what I had become, I was tired.

It all became too much for me to bear and at that moment it happened. I was blessed with the revelation that - because I did not gain this weight quickly, I was not going to lose it quickly. So why did I have this unrealistic expectation that it would magically fall off after two weeks because I ate salad for a week? The same time it took to get on me was probably going to be the same time it would possibly take to get off, if not longer.

Health Check Side Note:
Becoming overweight doesn't happen overnight, it happens over time, when the sustenance we take in by eating is not in balance with the energy we burn from being active.

Though I did not allow many photos of myself to be taken when I was at my heaviest of 195 pounds, I was able to provide two showing me at my heaviest of 195pd.

Me at 195 pounds holding my precious daughter

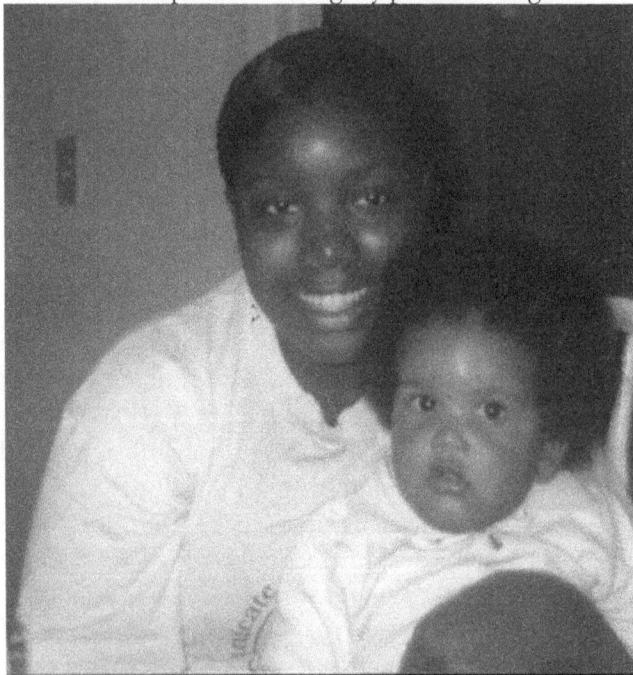

Chapter
2

THERE IS NO MAGIC PILL

There I was 5'2 weighing in at an overwhelming number of 195 pounds, battling a body image complex and several insecurities. I was so ashamed of what I had become. After gaining the weight I could barely stand to be in the presence of other women because I saw the beauty in them that I wished I saw in myself. I believed that I possessed no good looks. All I saw when I looked in the mirror; was ugliness, fat and a long list of things that were wrong with me.

I could not help but compare myself to the standard of beauty that was shown to me by the television and magazines. Never did I think that I was good enough. I was ashamed of myself and willingly allowed the weight to hinder me to the point where I didn't want to shop anymore, I stopped taking pictures, and the television became my only friend.

I was hurting, lost and lonely with the mindset of "*what*

man would give me a second glance?" I never felt good enough or pretty enough. Instead of seeking help I withdrew deeper inside myself and became even more angry and mean. I stopped socializing with my peers, and the television became my solace. I was a prisoner of hope with no clear direction to turn. Daily I wished that one day I would lose the weight so I could finally feel free to live. I walked with the mistaken impression that to be small was to be happy and free.

At a junction I stood. I wanted to lose the weight, yet I was still somewhat unwilling to do what was necessary to be fit and healthy. Contemplating my options, I began to think about my past actions and how I could do better in my present. I realized that five - almost six - years of my adult life were spent with me bemoaning my weight, constantly unhappy, and wishing for better.

The only bright light of joy I had was being with my daughter. However, I needed more. I wanted more. So I decided to do something about it. Moving forward I was determined not to allow another day pass without working towards becoming a better me.

Disgusted with myself for more reasons than one, but at that moment, for allowing myself to become a statistic of obesity in America I knew that something had to change. I was tired of being angry, I was tired of being unhappy, and most importantly I was tired of being a fat blob that was tipping against the scales of life. Was it not finally time to put forth some action?

Maybe all the extra weight would not have been so bad if

it just went strictly to my hips and butt. Unfortunately to my disappointment that was not the case, my weight went everywhere. I happened to have the female body type that weight looked absolutely hideous on, best described as an apple shape.

When I gained weight it went everywhere, my stomach, back, arms, thighs, breast, neck, and even my feet. I like apples but Lord knows I did not want to be shaped like one!

Health Check Side Note:
To help you better understand what I mean by apple shape provided below is a image, list and small description of the four most popular shapes used to describe the build of a woman:

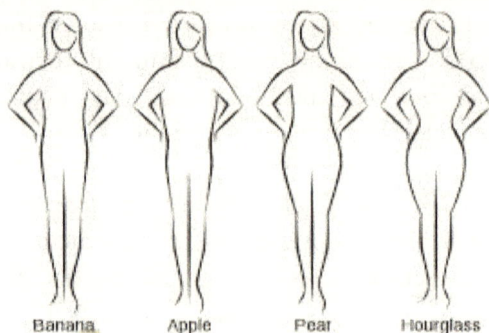

Banana   Apple   Pear   Hourglass

➢   Banana, straight, or I shape:

The waist measurement is less than 9 inches smaller than the hips and bust measurement. Body fat is distributed predominantly in the abdomen, butt, chest, and face. This overall fat distribution creates the typical straight shape.

➤ Apple or V shape:
Women that have broader shoulders compared to their hips. Apple shaped women tend to have slim legs and/or thighs, while the abdomen and chest look larger compared to the rest of the body. Fat is mainly distributed in the abdomen, chest, and face.

➤ Pear, spoon, bell, or A shape:
The hip measurement is greater than the bust measurement. The distribution of fat tends to deposit first in the buttocks, hips, and thighs. The women of this body type tend to have a (relatively) larger rear, thicker thighs, and a small bosom.

➤ Hourglass or X shape: The hip and bust are almost of equal size with a narrow waist. Body fat distribution tends to be around both the upper body and lower body. This body type enlarges the arms, chest, hips, and rear before other parts, such as the waist and upper abdomen.

(For more information visit)
http://www.calculator.net/body-type-calculator.html

******

Miserable I knew it was time to stop talking about losing weight and just be about it. With the decision made to take action, I slowly began taking the steps needed to ensure me a healthier body image. My first step was to stop making excuses.

In the past I constantly allowed myself to focus on the reasons why it was not possible for me to have a healthier lifestyle, instead of the real issue at hand, which was my unwillingness to stay any course of action let alone exercise.

My second step was to release the fear I had of being laughed at, talked about, or stared at. I was so big I was afraid to be seen doing anything physical. I thought people would laugh and judge me because I was a fat girl in the gym. Lastly I had to overcome my laziness: I never had any great desire to push myself beyond what was difficult, which continued to hinder any progress I tried to achieve.

START SOMEWHERE

For once in my life I was ready to attack and accomplish a goal. I wanted to lose weight. I was determined to lose weight. But three things seemed to be standing in my way: money, time, and childcare. I lacked the finances needed to join a gym, even if I could get the money to pay for a membership I did not have anyone to look after my daughter, and no way did I think it was possible for me to squeeze working out into my schedule.

With my old mentality of thinking there was no way I would have possibly been able to fit exercise into my tight agenda of working, eating, sleeping, and watching television. However, for once, something was different. I was different.

I was tired of the constant inner turmoil. Tired of the excuses, tired of being the fat sidekick, tired of hearing the whispers "what happened to her?" or "she used to be so...." and most of all tired of being the sister that got picked on and laughed at because I was no longer as pretty as my other sisters.

Determined to lose weight I decided to stop allowing the current inability I had to join a gym (or purchase exercise materiel/equipment) to continue being the deciding factor of my decisions. Though I did not have a lot going for me, what I did have was access to and free rein of the outdoors, which would cost me absolutely nothing to take advantage of it but time and energy.

As a result of my new way of thinking a plan began to take root into my heart. As simple as it seems now, I decided to take this weight loss journey one day at a time. I would no longer overwhelm myself with how much I had to lose but take it slow and prove to myself that I could work hard, that I could accomplish something, that there was more to me than struggle and lame excuses. Therefore, by changing my perspective I opened the doors to take the first steps needed to change my life.

In order for me to accomplish my goals, I had to brainstorm and identify the free time I did have available to work out. Due to the type of schedule I had in 2006 I did not have to be at work until 1215 in the afternoon. Which worked to my advantage and purpose for it allotted me the ability to drop my daughter of at school in the morning, leaving me a good two hours of free time.

Just that simply I found the kink in the chain and I decided to use at least one of those hours to exercise. So began my new routine: I dropped my daughter off at school, returned home, put on my workout clothes, went outdoors, and proceeded to walk around the neighborhood.

The first day was easy because it was new and exciting. I never had problems with first days - it was the fourth and fifth days that got me. By the second week of my physical activity I was tired and wanted to quit.

Consistency always seemed to be what kept me from succeeding in most things I started. Would I do what I had always done before and throw in the towel just because the going got a little tough? Or would I soldier on even after the excitement wore off?

Health Check Side Note:

Being a self-starter really sucks. There will be days when you will want to give up but you can't, just push through the pain, the excuses, and the desire to put it off until tomorrow. If you don't give up you will eventually break boundaries and achieve goals that you only once before could only talk or dream about.

▪▪

Though I did not want to use the two hours of freedom to work out, I pushed beyond the laziness by constantly reminding myself that this was something I wanted. Therefore I made the choice to keep pushing beyond my desire to quit by refusing to give up.

Health Check Antidote

Don't resent doing the exercise as if weight loss was not something you asked for. Are you not the one who said you were tired of being fat? Well act like it and exercise with joy and purpose. Yes, sometimes you will have to motivate yourself. I remember plenty of days I had to encourage and hype myself into action.

▪▪

EVERYTHING COUNTS

Eventually the positive change that was taking place in my personal life began to extend to my work habits. While at work, I decided not to shy away from anything that required the exertion of energy. For I knew that every time I moved was an opportunity to burn calories. Any potential pounds that I could get to melt away just from going about my daily activities was a added bonus.

As time went on I gained more confidence in my ability to succeed, so I decided to take a small financial leap by investing a little money into this weight loss endeavor, by purchasing a scale and a tape measure.

Boy was I rewarded by my efforts for I was pleasantly surprised by the loss of ten pounds. I was 185! Yes, that was still big but at least I was no longer five pounds shy of being 200 pounds. The way I saw it, any decrease in numbers created an increase in my faith and in my ability to succeed.

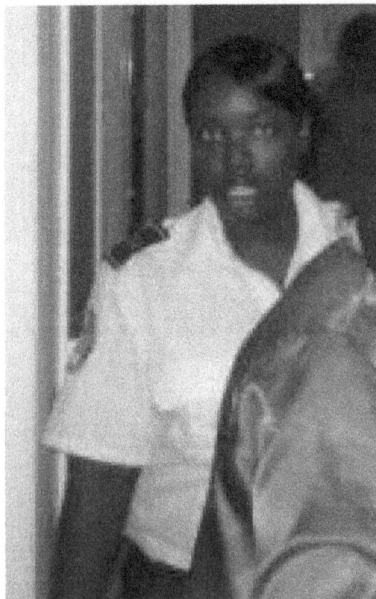

Ahlumba at 185

IT IS TIME

One year and twenty eight pounds later it was now time to increase my fitness efforts. I was consistently walking around the neighborhood for months, was no longer winded and I felt stronger. For that reason I believed I could now trust myself to up the ante. I was proud because I successfully stayed the course and remained dedicated to the goal I set.

Now it was time for me to increase my fitness goals and expectations. So I decided to throw caution to the wind and use the exercise center at my new job. It was now 2007 and I was employed by the City of Atlanta. On the fourth floor of City Hall (where I just so happened to work) was a fitness center available to all employees to use for free.

Of course, I never used it because: number one it was in plain sight of everyone to see; two I was embarrassed; and three time...I had no time to go over there. But I did have time, once again I failed to realize it. As long as I found time to eat, I had time to work-out, therefore I designated my lunch period as the time I would use to exercise.

LAUGH IT UP

The first day I decided to use the fourth floor gym at my work location was my introduction to many new things, however the elliptical was the most prevalent. That machine was challenging, hard, difficult, and exciting all at once. I remember my first time using it, initially I set the timer for ten minutes, but after barely a minute on it I knew that was a major mistake. As a result I reset the timer for the work-out to five minutes.

During my first work-out on the elliptical I was sweating profusely, I was out of breath and trying my darnedest to push beyond the pain. But when those five minutes were completed I was overjoyed. Overjoyed that the torture was over, and proud that I not only did it but successfully completed it. All I can remember thinking is how that was the hardest five minutes of my life.

After my initial shock over the intensity of the elliptical had passed, to the fourth floor gym I went three times a week. Where once my weight loss had become stagnate again the pounds began to decrease.

Just as I previously surmised people did see me; they stared, some laughed, and others picked at me. Some was good-natured laughter others was snidely done.

Health Check In
As you pursue your purpose you will encourage others. In the beginning it was just me and probably one other individual but as I consistently worked out more people began to follow.

✳ ✳ ✳ ✳ ✳

The naysayers and the supporters alike began to notice my weight loss. The nay-say-haters tried to use their authority to stop me from going, but the supporters would congratulate and ask me redundant questions such as...*You look good, what are you doing?* For which I would laugh good-naturedly and say *"you see me all the time I'm working out!"*

Me at 172

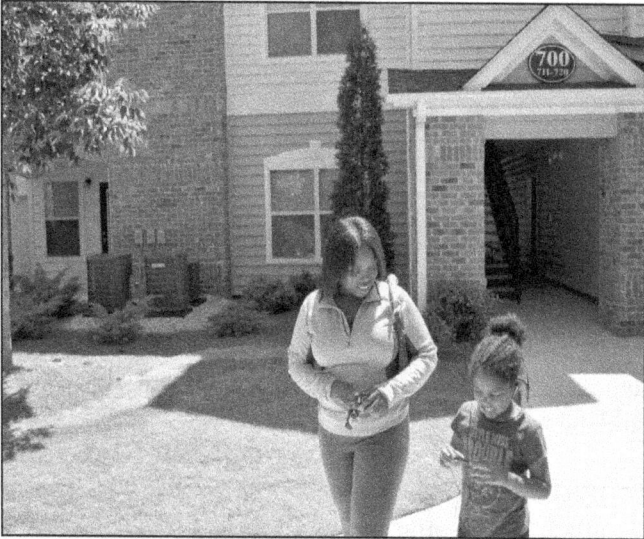

Me at 160

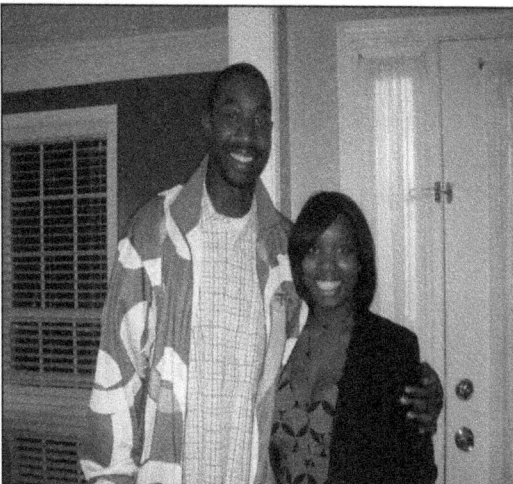

Health Check Side Note:
Seeing results is one of the most exciting things. If you don't give up
and stay persistent you will loss in turn win.

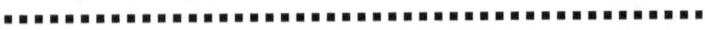

■■

SOMETIMES CHANGE IS A GOOD THING

This went on for almost year and I was at my whit's end (in a good way). There I was, 172 pounds when I first began working out at my job's gym (barely able to complete a five minute set) to working out almost an hour on my lunch break! I was truly blowing my mind. But of course things never go long periods of time without incurring some sort of set-back or change.

Eventually the powers that be made the decision to move me off site to an installation. Why? Why? Why did they have to do that? I was doing so well. I was losing all this weight but I knew all that would stop if I left City Hall because it was not possible for me to exercise at the fourth floor gym if I no longer had access to it during my lunch.

Once the word got out that I was leaving, coworkers began coming up to me inquiring how I was going to work out now that I was leaving. All I could do was shake my head and say, "*I don't know,*" but inside I was nervous and scared. I had a great routine, granted I hated my job, but the only enjoyment I received from that place was during the time I was able to work out. How was I going to exercise now?

Unbeknownst to me I had no reason to fret. The day I started at the new location I decided to map out an outdoor trail so that I could continue working out. However I did not use the trail immediately, because one of the guys at the new installation I was supporting, informed me that there was a YMCA no more than two minutes away from the shop - that had a workout facility and offered City of Atlanta employee discounts.

Excited, I wondered if I was really ready for such a big leap of commitment. Was I really ready to pay to work-out? Yes! I was. In the last two years I had grown so much. I had broken down so many walls that I never thought would come down. I was no longer that girl that was afraid to face the music.

Well, I joined that gym and stayed committed for almost two years. It was one of the best decisions

NO LONGER THE SAME GIRL

Before I knew it I was running; I was lifting weights; I was riding bikes and climbing mountains! Who was this girl? Exercise was like a drug, I could never get my fill of it or enough. It was fun and I was seeing results.

* * * * * *

Health Check Tip

It is imperative that you stay encouraged! I stayed encouraged by immersing myself in things that motivated me such as; The Biggest Loser, stories from the Joy Fit Club, weight loss blogs, and anything inspirational. Believe it or not I also enjoyed watching the weight loss infomercials. I took courage in their victories knowing that if they could achieve it so could I.

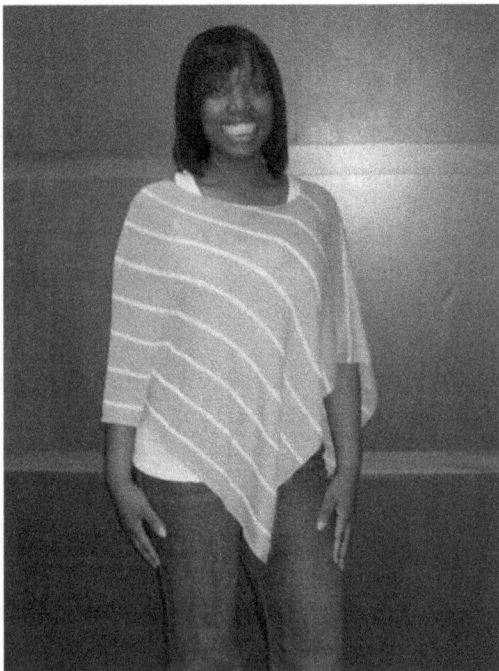

Feeling good in my Express size 8 jeans 150 pounds

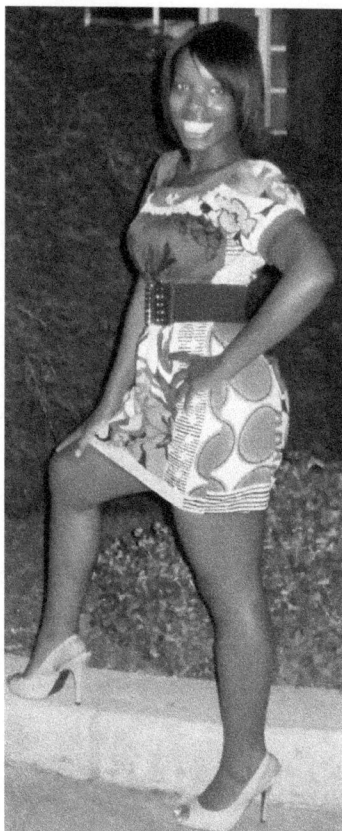

Fun evening out with the ladies.

Chapter
3

I CAN EAT & STILL LOSE WEIGHT

Exercise is good and important for it is one of the key elements to losing weight. But if exercise is the key then food would be the lock. For what good is a key if you have no door to open. Well, I loved good food and to this day still do.

Especially the things that are red flagged as a no-no. Such as bread, bread, and more bread, rice, pasta, fried anything...mainly chicken and how could I almost forget Chinese food. However eating all those yummy things without using some form of constraint is what originally got me into trouble.

If I thought getting my fat butt out there to walk was hard, changing my diet was no picnic whatsoever. I was tasked with the responsibility of learning how to curb my bad dieting while incorporating a form of healthy eating that worked best for my lifestyle. As a result of my lack of knowledge I felt compelled to do some research.

Health Check Side Note;

Find what works best for you. Every person is different whether exercising or consuming food. Just because counting calories worked for me does not mean it will work for you. It is imperative that you learn your body and work towards that end, not another.

■■

From the very beginning I knew that there were certain foods that I did not want to exclude from my daily diet. For if at any time my body felt like it was denied or restricted from any type of food, I would then immediately yearn for what I could not have.

That is why weight watchers stuck out to me. Not the point system but the calorie counting. With renewed confidence I took a leaf from their book and began researching what a safe attainable daily calorie intake was for someone my height and desired weight verses my current weight. After reading several health related articles I finally settled on a 1200-1500 calorie count diet. Of course to fluctuate (decrease or increase) based on my workouts and daily activities.

Health Check In:

Determining Your Calories

To lose weight, most people need to reduce the number of calories they get from food and beverages (energy IN) and increase their physical activity (energy OUT).
For a weight loss of 1–2 pounds per week, daily intake should be reduced by 500 to 1,000 calories.

In general the rule of thumb:

> ➢ *Eating plans that contain 1,000–1,200 calories each day will help most women lose weight safely.*

> ➢ *Eating plans that contain 1,200–1,600 calories each day are suitable for men and also may be appropriate for women who weigh 165 pounds or more or who exercise regularly.*

If you eat 1,600 calories a day but do not lose weight, then you may want to cut back to 1,200 - 1400 calories. If you are hungry, then you may want to boost your calories by 100 to 200 per day. Very low calorie diets of fewer than 800 calories per day should not be used unless you are being monitored by your doctor.

■ ■

Since I decided to go the route of counting calories I was therefore tasked with locating a fairly reputable calorie counter calculator. For which I found sparkpeople.com. Spark People had everything I needed. It offered me all the tools I was looking for with the added bonus of providing access to an online community that encouraged healthy living. I could track almost anything I consumed whether it was fast-food, normal food, beverages, or snacks.

STARTING YOUR DAY RIGHT

In the past I was a very inconsistent sporadic eater. There were many times I would not eat breakfast nor would I eat a proper lunch or dinner. Unaware of the harm l was doing to myself I withheld the proper nourishment from my body in turn hindering it from operating at its best. A typical day of eating for me looked similar to the following.

■■

Before Weight loss:

Breakfast:

➢ Nothing

➢ If I did eat it was dinner food such as baked chicken, rice with gravy, greens or peas, and juice or soda occasionally water

➢ Chinese Food

➢ Basically whatever was leftover from dinner from the previous night

Lunch:

➢ Hot wings, French fries, and soda

➢ Chinese food, shrimp fried rice, pepper steak, shrimp-egg-foo-young, and soda

➢ Hamburger, French fries, soda

Snacks:

➢ Potato Chips

➢ Candy Bars

➢ Soda

➢ Cake

➢ Brownies

Dinner:

➢ Pizza

➢ Chinese

➢ Whatever fast-food I had a taste for.

■■

AFTER WEIGHT LOSS

Breakfast:

➢ A Bowl of cereal and two boiled or scrambled eggs, with water

Lunch:

➢ Various types of meat wraps, lightly salted lays potato chips, two or three cookies (such as Oreos), and water

Snack:

➢ Fruit, such as banana, apple, pineapple, or grapes, and water

Dinner:

➢ Rice, Sautéed okra, fried fish, and water (My favorite evening meal)

■■

BREAKFAST ISN'T BAD AFTER ALL

Learning to eat breakfast daily was at first hard to grasp, but eventually I began to notice that eating properly had its positive effects. I was no longer starving when it was time for lunch, I had more energy in the morning, and I felt good. It amazed me that I could still eat the foods and snacks that I liked and still lose weight.

As my stomach got smaller it became easier for me to go without certain staple foods because I was not hungry. Even though I began to enjoy eating breakfast in the morning (just enough to get my metabolism going) hands down lunch was my favorite meal.

On the weekends I at times rewarded myself with something special like a bacon cheese burger with no fries or I would eat half of whatever meal I happened to be eating at the time that was high in fat, sodium, and calories to balance it out. Moderation was always key.

Health Check Side Note:
Starting Your Day Off Right...The benefits of eating breakfast:

> - *Provides energy*

> - *Allows for better focus*

> - *Helps to reduce crankiness*

> - *Gets your metabolism going allowing for optimum calorie burn*

> ➤ *Delaying your breakfast will cause your body to store calories in turn creating fat*

> ➤ *Prevents overeating*

■■■

Of course several occasions arose when I did not have time to prepare my meals ahead of time, and that is when all the discipline I garnered and information I learned earlier on about my body kicked in.

Health Check Tip:

You will have to learn to maintain and control your diet even at the most inopportune times. Maintaining your diet is like working out. It won't always be easy or convenient, but achieving anything great normally isn't.

■■■

Another key thing I have learned is that it is imperative that you lose weight the way you eat. Meaning, if you know you have no intention of taking bread out of your diet permanently then don't take it out while you are trying to lose weight because as soon as you add it back in you will gain back whatever you previously lost and possibly more.

31

I learned the hard way that not eating and skipping meals only hurt your body and hinders healthy habits. If your ultimate goal is to lose weight and be healthy then breakfast is an integral part of the process. Remember it is very important to the success of your weight loss to start your day off right by eating a hearty healthy meal.

By not eating breakfast you take the risk of:

➢ Slowing down your metabolism.

➢ Storing fat longer in your body.

➢ Overeating at your next meal.

➢ Weight gain.

WATER IS ESSENTIAL

I never thought my intake of water was a problem until I realized that I was not drinking enough of it. Since water has become my top source used to relieve my thirst I have noticed how it has helped to replenish and rejuvenate my body. Also I credit water for the clearness of my skin, the health of my hair, and the brightness of my smile.

Water was and still is one of the major factors involved in losing and maintaining my weight for that reason it is a must that I share some of the beneficial facts that I learned on how and why water should also be an important part of your weight-loss journey.

Why Water Is Important

✓ Initial weight loss is largely due to loss of water, and you need to drink an adequate amount of water in order to avoid dehydration.

✓ The process of burning calories requires an adequate supply of water in order to function efficiently; dehydration slows down the fat-burning process.

✓ Burning calories creates toxins and water plays a vital role in flushing them out of your body.

✓ Dehydration causes a decrease in blood level; a reduction in blood volume causes a reduction in the supply of oxygen to your muscles; and a reduction in the supply of oxygen to your muscles can make you feel tired.

✓ Water helps maintain muscle tone by assisting muscles in their ability to contract, and it lubricates your joints. Proper hydration can help reduce muscle and joint soreness when exercising.

✓ A healthy (weight loss) diet includes a good amount of fiber. But while fiber is normally helpful to your digestive system, without adequate fluids it can cause constipation instead of helping to eliminate it.

✓ Drinking water with a meal may make you feel full sooner and therefore satisfied thereby eating less. Note, however, that drinking water alone may not have this effect. In order to feel satiated (not hungry), our bodies need bulk, calories and nutrients.

Information bullets were attained from
http://www.caloriesperhour.com/tutorial_water.php

Here is some additional information to help you determine how much water is enough.

How much water you actually need depends on your weight, level of activity, the temperature or humidity of your environment, and your diet. Your diet makes a difference because if you eat plenty of water-dense foods like fruits and vegetables your need to drink as much water will be diminished.

You can also do some research, use a calculator or a measuring cup if you like, however your body is pretty good at letting you know the right amount to drink. When you drink enough water, your urine will usually be pale yellow, though vitamin supplements and antibiotics can discolor it. On the other hand, you shouldn't need to run to the bathroom too frequently. When in doubt, drink a little more.

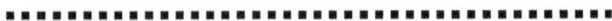

■■

Health Check Side Note
Tips for heart healthy eating:

1. *Eat less saturated and* trans *fat. Stay away from fatty meats, fried foods, cakes, and cookies.*

2. *Cut down on sodium (salt). Look for the low-sodium or "no salt added" types of canned soups, vegetables, snack foods, and lunch meats.*

3. *Get more fiber. Fiber is in vegetables, fruits, and whole grains.*

Provided below are some additional heart healthy, energy boosting shopping list ideas to help get you started:

Vegetables and Fruits

➢ Fresh vegetables such as tomatoes, cabbage, broccoli, and spinach
➢ Leafy greens for salads
➢ Canned vegetables low in sodium (salt)
➢ Frozen vegetables without added butter or sauces
➢ Fresh fruits such as berries, apples, oranges, bananas, pears, and peaches
➢ Canned fruit in 100% juice, not syrup
➢ Frozen or dried fruit (unsweetened)

Milk and Milk Products

It is suggested that you purchase fat-free milk, low-fat

milk, or soy products with added calcium. However my opinion is to purchase the best milk products for you and your family.

- ➢ Fat-free or low-fat (1%, 2% or whole) milk
- ➢ Fat-free or low-fat yogurt
- ➢ Cheese (3 grams of fat or less per serving)

Breads, Cereals, and Grains

For products with more than one ingredient, make sure whole wheat or another whole grain is listed first.

- ➢ 100% whole-wheat bread
- ➢ Whole-grain breakfast cereals like oatmeal
- ➢ Whole grains such as brown or wild rice, barley, and bulgur
- ➢ Whole-wheat or whole-grain pasta

Meat, Beans, Eggs, and Nuts

Choose lean cuts of meat and other foods with protein.

- ➢ Seafood, including fish and shellfish
- ➢ Chicken and turkey breast without skin
- ➢ Pork: leg, shoulder, tenderloin
- ➢ Beef: round, sirloin, tenderloin, extra lean ground beef
- ➢ Beans, lentils, and peas
- ➢ Eggs
- ➢ Nuts and seeds

Fats and Oils

Cut back on saturated fat and look for products with no trans fats. However I still use good old fashion butter.

- ➢ Margarine and spreads (soft, tub, or liquid) with no trans fats
- ➢ Vegetable oil (canola, olive, peanut, or sesame)
- ➢ Non-stick cooking spray
- ➢ Light or fat-free salad dressing and mayonnaise

For additional information about heart healthy foods and how they benefit your body visit healthfinder.gov.

CHAPTER
4

ONE SIZE HEALTHY

"WOW! I did it, I really did it." I looked in the mirror and finally liked what I saw! For six years I was the unhappy fat girl who hated to see her own image in any mirror. Therefore after I lost the weight I was not surprised by my initial reactions to it. Whenever I caught a glimpse of myself in a mirror I would pause in awe surprise, for the image I had grown used to seeing was no longer there.

In its place was a face and body that I had long forgotten. As a result I could not resist the urge I had to stare at my own reflection with giddy appreciation. For it was in those moments that I felt as if I was seeing myself for the first time in a very long time.

It took me over two years to lose 65 pounds. I know what you are thinking, "Two years, that's a long time!" Yes, it is long, but I was not in a race with anyone. For as long as I can remember I took the microwave approach to things, thirty seconds then done. This however was not so quickly remedied for it was my life that hung in the balance. I was on a journey of self love, self discovery, forgiveness and healing. It was not until I looked in the mirror and saw the transition of me that I realized it to be. My journey was, and still is, a daily walk and I am totally fine with pacing myself.

For over five years all I did was complain and talk about my weight. It was not until I created a plan of attack and put it into action that I began to not only see my outer transform but the persona of my inner self began to change for the better.

In your journey to becoming one size healthier, it is imperative that you create a plan and make it clear. From childhood, to the age of twenty, I took for granted that I would be small for my entire life. I literally talked negatively about what I eventually became.

It took me to gain sixty-five, very unattractive pounds, for me to find out what kind of metal I was made of. This weight loss journey was not a walk in the park, many times I almost crumbled from the pressure that I put on myself, but God always strengthened me. Slowly I began to see the results I worked so hard to achieve and the release of a better temperament .

In this portion of the book I encourage you to map out your own weight loss plan of attack.

<u>My Plan Of Attack</u>

1). Why do you want to lose weight?

_____

_____

_____

_____

_____

_____

_____

_____

_____

_____

_____

_____

_____

2). How much weight would you like to lose?

_____

_____

_____

_____

3). What is your current diet like?

_____

_____

_____

_____

4). What type of exercise routine will you initiate?

_____

_____

_____

_____

5). What challenges will you have to overcome?

_____

_____

_____

_____

6). When will you begin your weight loss journey?

_____

_____

_____

_____

BEFORE WEIGHT LOSS

1). What is your start weight? _____

2). Be sure to take a "Before" photo if you have not already.

Place Photo

Place Photo

Here

Here

3). Take your Measurements! There will be times when the scale will not move but you would have lost inches.

Before measurements

✓ Neck: _____

✓ Bust: _____

✓ Waist: _____

✓ Thigh: _____

✓ Arms: _____

After Measurements

✓ Neck: _____

✓ Bust:: _____

✓ Waist: _____

✓ Thigh: _____

✓ Arms: _____

ONE SIZE HEALTHY

Chapter
5

WIPE-OUT THE EXCUSES

By now you are probably thinking, "She's right…but…" There is no "but" just "do" by doing what you can with the means that you have now. No matter what you see as a hindrance or an obstacle, I am here to inform you that there is always a way when there is a will.

Before I made the decision to actually be about the business of changing my life - by losing all that excess - weight I had more excuses than a little bit. I truly believed that it was not possible for me to achieve the goal of being healthier by way of exercising and eating properly.

Yet by the grace of God, faith, persistence, inspiration, hard work, and time I was able to go from weighing one hundred and ninety five pounds to weighing one hundred and thirty pounds.

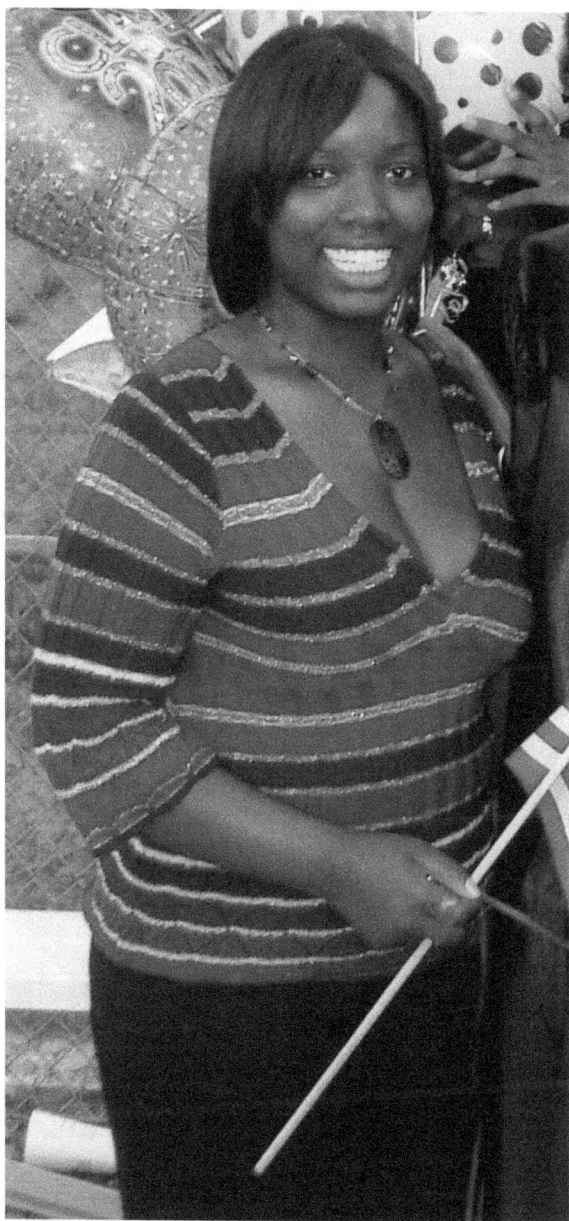

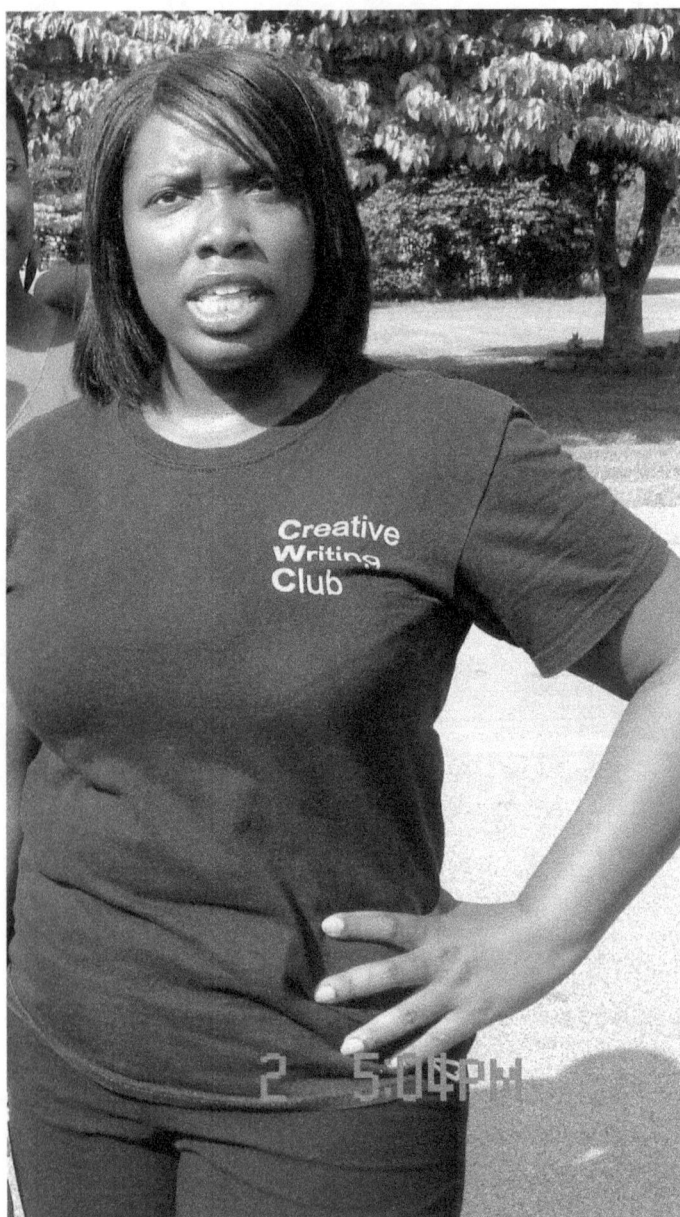

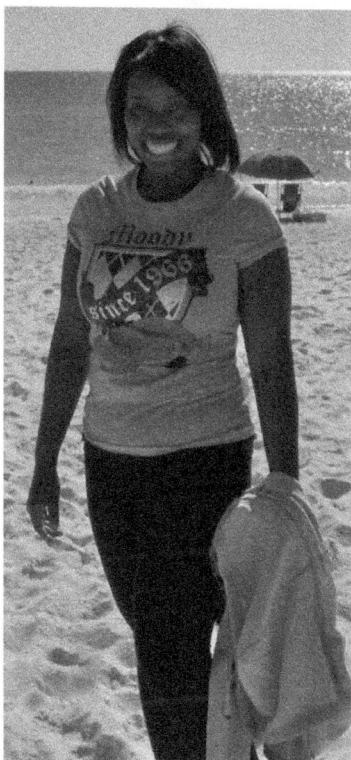

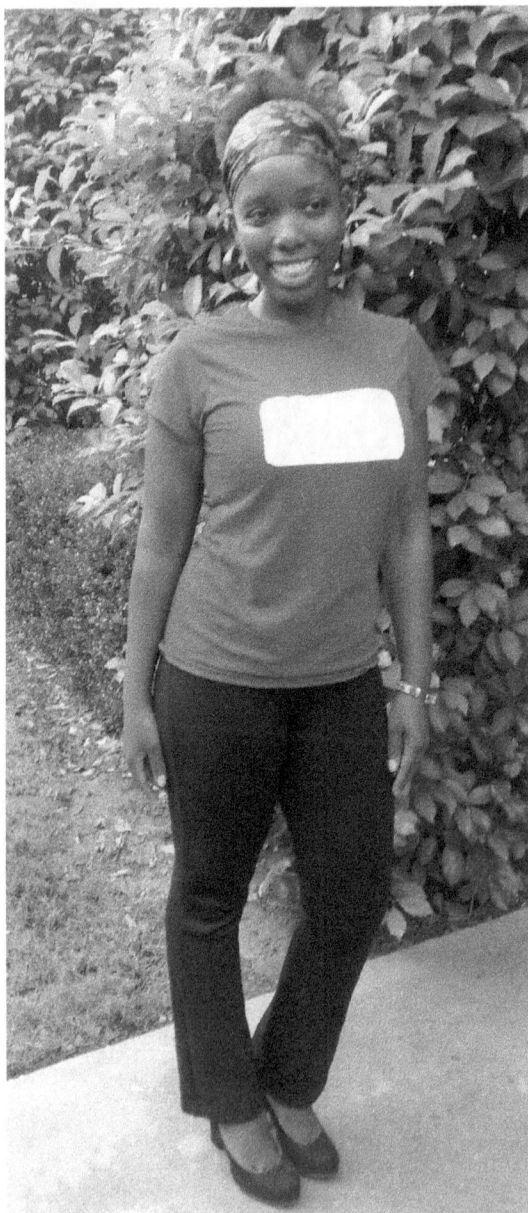

Don't let anything stop you from achieving your dream, vision, or goal; not even your own reasoning. Below I provide a list of some of my most common excuses:

1. **No money:** The traditional route that most think of when they first decide to lose the weight is to gain membership at an gym, join a boot camp, or purchase weight loss paraphernalia (such as: workout DVD's, fitness machines, fitness gadgets).

    Though those things are wonderful assets to have access to, it should not be the factor that stops you from doing it. Why? Because as long as there are parks, the outdoors, trails, mountains, tracks, and open fields it allows you to get started for free. When you are a beginner it is important to start from somewhere; don't jump into the big waters until you have proven to yourself that you can swim.

2. **No Time or Energy:** Time is the essential component that runs our day. We judge our daily list of activities by the amount of free time we are able to siphon. One of my favorite things to say to anyone who would listen was, "I want to work-out but I don't have any time." It was not until I made an evaluation of how my time was spent, that I noticed all the gaps in my schedule that

indeed did allow free opportunities to exercise.

I could wake up an hour earlier before it was time to get up; use my lunch break or 15 minute breaks; instead of lounging on the couch or bed while watching television use that time to exercise.

I knew my weakness, I had a lack of follow through on certain things. No matter how many times I said that I would work out after I got off of work it was not going to happen. I was more alert in the mornings and afternoons, so to get the most out of that energy, I decided to fit my workouts in during my lunch period.

Health Check Tip:

It is imperative that you be honest with yourself, if you know that you are normally tired when you get off work and you don't have the self-discipline to push yourself to follow through, then by all means do not make plans to work-out during that period of the day. Don't set yourself up for failure.

3. **Lack of Discipline:** How many times have you said, *I need to work out but I don't feel like it?* That same laziness is the reason why you are fat now and will remain that way until you change by consistently getting up by way of exerting the action needed to achieve your goal.

4. **No Babysitter:** I was very protective of my one

and only child; so, whenever it came time for me to commit to something I would say, "I can't because I don't have anyone to watch Aniyla." It was not until I realized that it was better to participate in activities that were child-friendly that I stopped allowing that excuse to stop me.

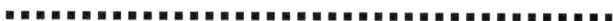

■■

Today chose to replace those washed-out excuses with some wonderful benefits of why exercise and good health is a necessity not a luxury:

- ✓ Improves eating habits

- ✓ Lowers risk of high blood pressure and diabetes

- ✓ Strengthens your heart

- ✓ Helps to reduce stress

- ✓ Builds self esteem

- ✓ Boost Immune system

- ✓ Causes weight loss

Overcoming excuses is not an easy feat, but eventually

you will have to face yourself in the mirror and ask, "Who am I really fooling?" In my opinion, the only way to remain healthy is to: build good eating habits, instill control, and most importantly maintain a regimen of exercise or fun active activities.

Health Check Side Note:

Here are some tips on how to be physically active without having to spend any money from the National Institute on Aging, National Institutes of Health, U.S. Department of Health & Human Services

- ✓ Get some exercise and have fun with friends while you walk the entire mall.

- ✓ Get your garden or yard in shape, and you'll shape up, too.

- ✓ Make your own weights from household items such as plastic, milk jugs filled with sand or water, bags of rice, soup cans, or bottles of water.

- ✓ Rather than driving, walk when doing errands. In your community

- ✓ Try out free demonstration exercise classes at your local center or fitness center

- ✓ Participate in community-sponsored fun runs or walks.

- ✓ Join a kickball or softball league that plays at your

community center.

✓ Go for a hike in a park.

✓ Learn about trees and plants while exploring a local arboretum.

✓ Help your community by participating in a stream clean-up effort.

All year round

✓ Borrow or use your own bicycle and ride around the neighborhood to admire the spring flowers.

✓ Play an early-morning tennis match at your community courts in the summer.

✓ Jog through the park and breathe in the crisp air.

Chapter 6

IT'S A DAILY WALK

Losing the weight is just the beginning, as in anything there is up keep. You would not expect to be able to bathe once and never touch water again, to get your hair done just to believe that you don't have to tie it up at night, to purchase a car and never get an oil change. Everything requires some form of maintenance.

After I made it to the size and weight that I was happy with I then began to loosen the reins of my work out just a little because I was no longer trying to lose weight but maintain it. I realized, and accepted, that I was not one of those individuals that had the metabolism of an animal which enabled them to eat anything and gain nothing.

I knew that for the rest of my life I would have to remain active in some form. It was important to be as mindful as I could possibly be when it came to what I put into my mouth.

Accept the fact that your weight will fluctuate; for that reason be sure to have a number in mind that you are comfortable with. For me it was five pounds. On average I weighed 133 pounds, so I told myself that if I ever got to 138 it would be time to buckle down - because I knew that I did not want to go pass my high end weight of 138.

No it won't always be easy but if you refuse to focus on the scale and the constraints of deadlines (we at times put on ourselves) you will free yourself to embark on a journey that is not only life changing but fun. Don't beat yourself up because of goals you have yet to reach. Here are some tips and fun ways to incorporate activity into your daily routine to help keep you moving.

I. Make Time

- Identify free times. Keep track of your daily activities for one week. Pick two 30 time slots you could use for family activity time.

- Add physical activity to your daily routine. For example, walk or ride your bike to work or a friend's house, walk the dog with your child(ren), exercise while you watch TV, or park farther away from your destination.

- Try to walk, jog, or swim during your lunch hour, or take fitness breaks instead of coffee breaks. Try doing something active after dinner with your family, or on weekends.

- Check out activities requiring little time. Try walking, jogging, or stair climbing.

II. Bring Others Into It
- Ask friends and family to support your efforts.

- Invite them to be active with you.

- Set up a party or other social event with activities that get people moving, like dancing or having a jump rope contest.

- Exercise with friends.

- Play with your kids or ask them to join you for an exercise video or fitness game.

- Develop new friendships with physically active people. Join a group, such as the YMCA or a hiking club.

III. Energize Yourself
- Plan to be active at times in the day or week when you feel you have a lot of energy.

- Convince yourself that if you give it a chance, physical activity will increase your energy level—then try it.

IV. Stay Motivated
- Plan ahead. Make physical activity a regular part

of your family's schedule. Write it on a family activity calendar.

- Join an exercise group or class. Sign your children up for community sports teams or lessons.

- Pick activities requiring no new skills, such as walking or climbing stairs.

- Exercise with friends who are at the same skill level as you are. Create opportunities for your children to be active with friends.

V. Build New Skills
- Find a friend who can teach you new skills.

- Take a class to develop new skills and enroll your children in classes too, such as swimming, dancing, or tennis.

VI. Use Available Resources
- Select activities that don't need costly sports gear, such as walking, jogging, jumping rope, or doing push-ups.

- Identify cheap, local resources in your area, such as programs through your community center, park or recreation group, or worksite.

VII. Make the Most of All Conditions
- Develop a set of activities for you and your family that are always available regardless of weather,

such as indoor cycling, indoor swimming, stair climbing, rope skipping, mall walking, dancing, and active games that you can play indoors.

- When the weather is nice, try outdoor swimming, jogging, walking, or tennis.

******

For over five years of my life I was less than a shell of what I was created to be. I hid behind excuses, fear, doubt, and self-abuse; which eventually brought to the forefront several insecurities I never knew resided in me.

I am well aquatinted with your struggle for I encounter it every day. It is up to you to make the choice to change your tomorrow by taking some better steps today. Do what you can with what you have and as you progress you will see the increase of opportunities to expand your efforts.

THE CLIMB

I liken this journey that you will embark on to climbing a mountain. Recently, I started going back to Stone Mountain Park to climb the mountain...those of you who are familiar with the park know that for the first timer it's a fairly arduous hike - one mile up one mile down totaling two miles round trip. Well, on this particular day, I was struck by how at the bottom of the mountain (where you begin your journey) there are several people who start with you; friends, family, coworkers, even strangers. Everyone is happy, taking pictures and eager to get their journey started...the excitement is palpable.

The the journey begins filled with energy most start off strong, eager, and excited about the challenge. A quarter mile in you get a few complainers who are not used to pushing themselves, so eventually they fall back because they are tired and did not expect it to take this long.

Eventually the half mile mark is reached (the resting post). At this point you get to see several people who decide to postpone their journey for awhile longer, or even worse they make the decision to give up until later.

Almost there you hit the 3/4 mile marker and realize there is practically no one around to share your struggles, fears, pain, uncertainties, or triumphs. That's when it really hits you that almost everyone you started with either gave up, stopped, or slowed down. However the one that decides to keep going even in the face of bleakness will be rewarded with reaching the top.

Sometimes to achieve your goal you will have to press forward on your own. Yes instances will arise when you become lonely, tired, a little lost, and at times confused but if you persist you will come into the knowledge that to reach your destination sacrifices must be made. Be bold and choose life, purpose, and fulfillment.

Don't pursue instant gratification - pursue your passion - for therein lies your purpose. Open your spectrum of thought. No matter what gets in your way or how long it takes never give up on your Dream, Vision, or Goal.

Chapter
7

THE UGLY TRUTH

The reality of my ongoing journey to be physically, spiritually, mentally, and financially healthy is that I faltered, I raged, I feared, and at times I have wanted to give up. However my Lord God - and the passion for purpose He has given me - would not allow me to remain defeated.

I am learning that without the dark storms (that at times weather our life) how could we ever appreciate the bright beauty of a new day? What began as a means to just look good turned into a revelation to realization of purpose. It was not just physical fitness that I was in need of but mental peace and self acceptance.

This journey that you are about to embark on, will in no way be easy, stress free, or without some level of difficulty; however it is imperative that you do not allow the doubts created by the negative attacks you will encounter hinder you from reaching your destiny.

UGLY TRUTH POINTERS:

Self Starting Is A Monster Of A Task!
➢ What was a breeze yesterday sometimes becomes a struggle today. The only way you will see any results in your life is to consistently take the steps needed to make it happen. Time is priceless yet we carelessly use it without ever making any real deposits to ensure the future success of our endeavors.

Be Enslaved To Nothing!
➢ When you are desperate for something you then become a ripe target for the picking. Be enslaved to nothing.

Never Enough!
➢ I never feel like I'm doing enough. *I'm not writing enough, not aggressive enough, not bold enough, not making enough, not praying enough, and at times not good enough.* When you begin to doubt your ability, you then give room for "fear" to attack, destroy, and tear down every dream vision or goal you ever hoped to accomplish in life.

Fear!
➢ Don't let fear stop you from attaining victory! Whatever you desire, dream of, or envision for your life will remain a figment of thought in your mind until you choose to work it out by way of

walking it out with action.

Desperation!
> ➢ Everything that looks good isn't good. Anything that is worth having will take time and hard work. There is no easy route to long lasting success, so beware of "get what you want quick schemes."

Be Free
> ➢ Never pretend to be anything other than who you are. Set your own standard of expectation, for perfection was only obtained by one.

Tribulation Will Come
> ➢ Could you imagine dreaming a dream; wanting and believing in it so deeply that you willingly go through the pain of tribulation, desolation, and loss just to obtain that dream you dreamed?

> Sometimes you will have to endure the chastisement of men and women alike, just to obtain what was denied you. Fight for what you believe in by standing resolute and unmoving for opposition will always arise however it is your responsibility to endure through it. No matter how long it takes never give up. No matter how many times you fall – always get back up.

Mental Stability
> ➢ Physical health is important; however, you must not allow your mental health to fall by the wayside. The quietness of meditation replenishes

and gives room for the Lord to not only speak but for you to finally hear Him.

Sometimes we get so lost in the noise of the world, life difficulties, and the hopes of our aspirations that we inadvertently lose our way. Remember it is God that continues to constantly provide you with the strength needed to keep going when all you want to do is throw in the towel.

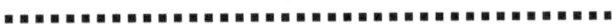

■■

NEVER GIVE UP

In closing, I implore you to be prepared by realizing that any goal you hope to achieve will not be brought to light without bearing some kind of difficulty. Even so, remain encouraged for God is able to carry out his purpose in your life bigger than you dared to hope for or even imagined!

Therefore don't ever let fear stop you from finding out whether or not something is an option or a possibility. Be it weight loss, a desire to further your education, a new career path, the possibility of a new relationship, or the daring to pursue a lifelong dream.

Be bold and take the leap or forever live in what could have been. Be dedicated to your choice by committing to the pursuit and attainment of your dream, instead of the reasons it cannot be done.

Just like you, I constantly strive to burst through the walls of containment and mediocrity that has been imposed upon me. But unlike many I am willing to fall and get back up again, for it is in the falling that you see a clearer direction, therefore realizing the strength of your character and clarity of purpose.

The only limitation we have is the one we create! If you have a will, I dare you not to make a way.

Today have the faith to believe, the boldness to take a chance, the tenacity to hold on, the endurance to last, and the confidence in yourself that your dream can become a reality.

One More Thought Before You Go

I looked in the mirror and I saw me
I was no longer the fat me but the pretty me
Now I would be happy
Now I would be free
But boy was I surprised
When that did not happen initially
See I thought that having a better outer
Would change my inner
When it was the transformation of my inner
That truly allowed me to see
That the beauty I failed to notice was already in me

~ Ahlumba

ABOUT THE AUTHOR

Ahlumba Harris a high school dropout, a college dropout, and a single mother of one who had the fortitude to search for and obtain more despite the mediocrity that tried to contain her. Just like you she constantly seeks to improve her physical, spiritual, and financial wellbeing for she is in a journey to reach her destiny...

INSPIRED2PROSPER INTERNATIONAL, LLC

GET THE APP

Have your daily Cup of Jo at the touch of your fingertips! Download the free app *'Morning Cup of Jo'* from the Google Play store today!

SHARE YOUR STORY WITH US

Have you obtained some personal success? Why not share it with us? Don't worry know success is ever to small to share, we want to celebrate with you.

If you have any questions, concerns, or inspiring words, please feel free to contact us at:
WWW.INSPIRED2PROSPER.COM
CONTACTUS@INSPIRED2PROSPER.COM

IF YOU WOULD LIKE MORE INFO ABOUT I2P
VISIT:
WWW.INSPIRED2PROSPER.COM
WWW.AHLUMBA.COM

YOU CAN ALSO LIKE AHLUMBA'S PAGES ON FACEBOOK:
WWW.FACEBOOK.COM/INSPIRED2PROSPER
WWW.FACEBOOK.COM/AHLUMBAH

OTHER BOOKS BY AHLUMBA HARRIS

Inspired2Prosper
Morning Cup of Jo

Coming Soon:
"Letters From a Desperate Heart"